Lynda AOUDIA

BI-RADS ultrasound glossary

Lynda AOUDIA

BI-RADS ultrasound glossary

step by step to classification

ScienciaScripts

Cover image: www.ingimage.com

This book is a translation from the original published under ISBN 978-620-6-71381-4.

Publisher:
Sciencia Scripts
is a trademark of
Dodo Books Indian Ocean Ltd. and OmniScriptum S.R.L publishing group

120 High Road, East Finchley, London, N2 9ED, United Kingdom
Str. Armeneasca 28/1, office 1, Chisinau MD-2012, Republic of Moldova, Europe
Managing Directors: Ieva Konstantinova, Victoria Ursu
info@omniscriptum.com

Printed at: see last page
ISBN: 978-620-8-56446-9

Contents

Foreword

Since 1993, the American College of Radiology (ACR) has published the BI-RADS "Breast Imaging-Reporting and Data System", which provides an accurate description of mammographic abnormalities, a detailed glossary of terms and a precise mammographic report including evaluation categories. As with mammography, an ultrasound BI-RADS lexicon was developed in 2003, at the same time as the 4th edition of the mammography BI-RADS, in order to standardise the characterisation of ultrasound lesions. The latest American version of the BI-RADS was published by the ACR in 2013, entitled BI-RADS® Atlas.

In this book, each term in the BI-RADS lexicon will be explained in detail, with the help of rich iconography, which will lead us to the BI-RADS classification of lesions and subsequently determine the appropriate management.

Professor Lynda AOUDIA

Introduction

The BI-RADS (Breast Imaging Reporting and Data System) developed by the American College of Radiology (ACR) in collaboration with other organisations, such as the Food and Drug Administration (FDA) and the National Cancer Institute. The initial aim of this tool was to improve the quality of breast cancer screening campaigns, by standardising mammography reports using a common lexicon, resulting in appropriate action and easier follow-up. This classification has a number of advantages, including guiding the radiologist in describing mammographic abnormalities by trying to reduce inter-observer discrepancies and standardising descriptive terms, resulting in the most reproducible classification possible and appropriate action to be taken.

As with mammography, an ultrasound BI-RADS lexicon was developed in 2003, at the same time as the 4th edition of the mammography BI-RADS, in order to standardise the characterisation of ultrasound lesions. The latest American version of the BI-RADS was published by the ACR in 2013, entitled BI-RADS® Atlas [1].

This assessment is based on a certain number of criteria (shape, contours, interface, orientation in relation to the skin, echogenicity, posterior acoustic signs, vascularity and hardness), according to which the anomalies will be classified in one of the five categories of the ACR BI-RADS lexicon according to the degree of suspicion of malignancy, which will enable us to propose appropriate management [1] (table 1).

Table 1. Bi-RADS® ultrasound assessment categories	
BI-RADS 0	Incomplete assessment, requiring further tests.
BI-RADS 1	Examination considered strictly normal
BI-RADS 2	Benign lesion(s): Simple cysts, intra-mammary lymph nodes, breast implants, stable post-surgical changes, probable stable fibroadenomas.
BI-RADS 3	Anomaly probably benign. Suggestion of short-term surveillance. For example: solid masses with a circumscribed outline, oval, parallel orientation (probable fibroadenoma), complicated cysts that cannot be palpated, clusters of microcysts.
BI-RADS 4	Suspicious abnormality, with a probability of malignancy of between 2 and 95%, requiring histological analysis. 4a = low probability > 2% to < 10%, 4b = moderate probability 10% to < 50%, 4c = high probability > 50 to < 95%.
BI-RADS 5	Highly suspicious abnormality, with > 95% probability of malignancy, requiring surgical removal.
BI-RADS 6	Known histological result: proven malignancy.

CHAPTER I

Anatomical reminder

1. Breast anatomy

The breast is a globular organ occupying the anterior-superior part of the thorax. It is located above the pectoralis muscle, which provides support [2]. It is mainly made up of a mammary gland, supporting connective tissue and adipose tissue, all covered by the skin. The apex of the breast is represented by the nipple surrounded by the areola (fig. 1). It is made up of around fifteen main milk ducts, each delimiting a lobe. The milk ducts open into the nipple at the level of the milk pores, after dilating slightly to form a lactiferous sinus.

Thin fibrous septa separate the lobes, extending into the dermis at the anterior surface of the gland to form Cooper's ligaments, which form Duret's ridges (fig. 1).

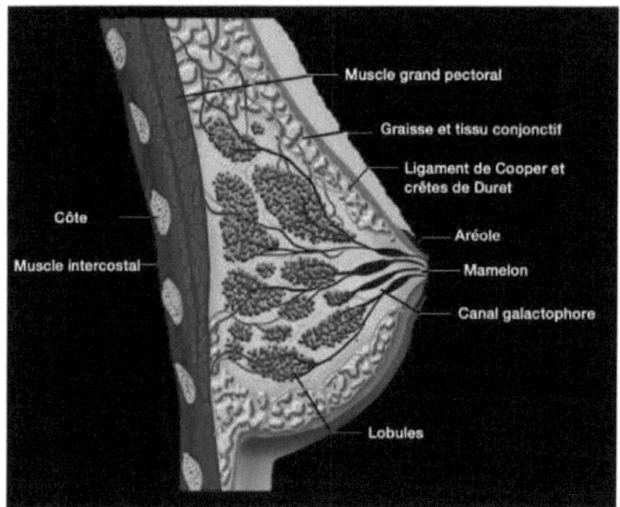

Fig. 1 Anatomical structure of the breast.

2. Galactophoric tree

The breast is made up of around fifteen main milk ducts, ending in a nipple pore. These main ducts, after a dilatation known as the lactiferous sinus, branch off into secondary ducts of medium and small calibre up to the Ductulo-Lobular Terminal Unit (DLTU).

This UDTL consists of a terminal extra- and intra-lobular galactophore and a lobule made up around ten alveoli called acini. The UDTL is embedded in a loose connective tissue known as pallial tissue. All of this tissue is surrounded by adipose tissue (fig. 2).

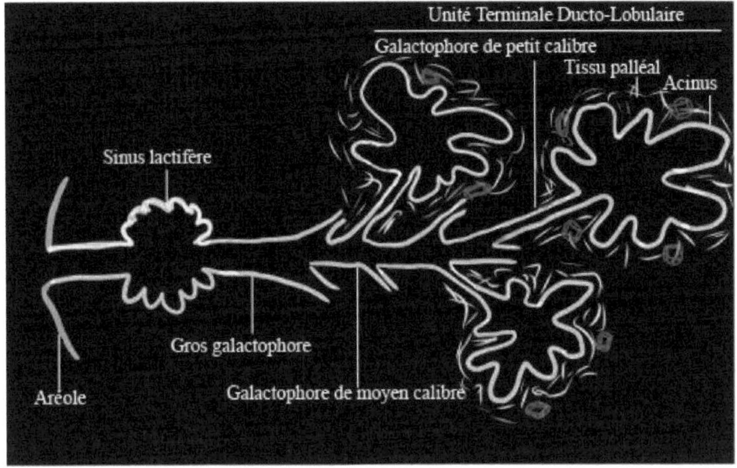

Fig. 2: Diagram of the galactophoric tree.

CHAPTER II

Histological reminder

The whole of the galactophoric tree is made up of a double layer of cells resting on a basal membrane in direct contact with the blood vessels (fig. 3): - an inner layer made up of cylindrical epithelial cells responsible for the milk secretory function.

- an outer layer made up of myoepithelial cells responsible for contraction.

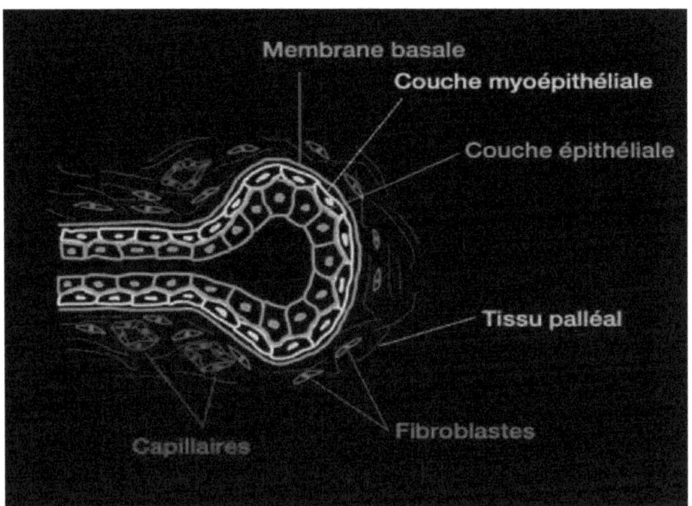

Fig. 3: Histological diagram of acinar constituents.

3. Ultrasound

Ultrasound is an accessible, non-irradiating and inexpensive imaging technique. It can be used as a complement to mammography, improve lesion detection, particularly in dense breasts, and to characterise lesions, in particular to differentiate between solid and cystic lesions, and to take samples [3].

Breast ultrasound is performed with a high-frequency probe, usually between 9 and 15 MHz, which provides good contrast and spatial resolution [4]. There are several ultrasound modes.

3.1. Mode B

This is the first technique used in breast ultrasound . Ultrasound waves are emitted and collected by the probe, at the same frequency, in a single direction. They are combined to create a 2D image of the breast on a greyscale [5]. This technique allows structures to be differentiated on the basis of the acoustic and mechanical properties of the tissue. This B-mode has a number of weaknesses, including inconsistent optimal resolution and artefacts that can degrade image quality [6] (fig. 4).

3.2. Harmonic mode

It is linked to the non-linear behaviour of breast tissue in relation to ultrasound. As the ultrasound wave propagates through breast tissue, it undergoes progressive distortion of the shape of the ultrasound pulse, creating harmonic frequencies which are multiples of the emission frequency [7-9]. Once the initial signal has been filtered, the harmonic signal is used to reconstruct the image. This technique improves the contrast of ultrasound images, particularly for cysts with "thick contents" or complicated cysts, which show internal echoes in B mode, in harmonic mode they appear anechoic [10] (fig. 4).

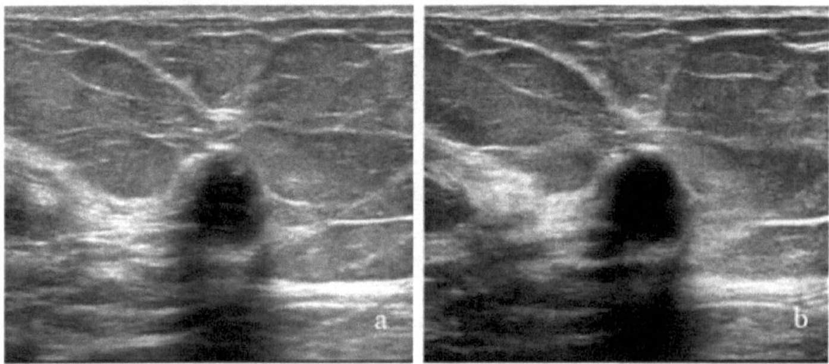

Fig. 4: Harmonic mode (a) B-mode ultrasound. Hypoechoic mass, (b) Harmonic mode ultrasound. Anechoic cystic mass with thickened wall. Histology. Histology: remodelled cyst.

3.3. Composite mode (Compound)

Two types of composite, frequency composite (several different frequencies of ultrasound emission are used to reconstruct the final image), and spatial composite (several angles of ultrasound emission are used and combined into a single composite image). This technique makes it possible to limit artefacts, improve analysis of lesion contours, better define the internal echostructure of masses and detect small lesions [11] (fig. 5). It also allows better detection of intra-lesional calcifications [12]. On the other hand, posterior ultrasound changes are attenuated [13].

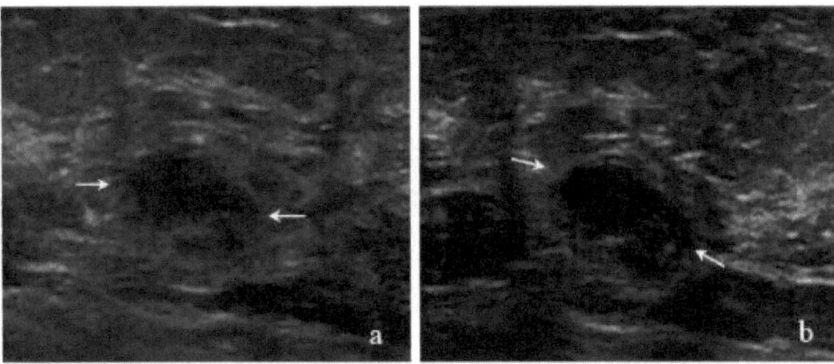

Fig. 5. composite mode. (a) B-mode ultrasound. Hypoechoic mass with indistinct contours, (b) Composite mode ultrasound. Hypoechoic, circumscribed mass. Histology: Adenofibroma.

It is used to detect tumour angiogenesis. Malignant lesions are generally more vascularised than benign lesions, with an abnormal, irregular appearance of the vessels. Detection and analysis of the spectrum of these vessels requires a probe of at least 10 MHz and a rigorous ultrasound technique (adjusting the focal length, reducing the overall gain, adapting the size of the Doppler boot, filtering to the minimum 10 in order to analyse the low frequencies, no pressure on the breast to avoid obliteration of the small vessels) [14, 15].

Energy Doppler has a better sensitivity to slow flows, but is more sensitive to artefacts [13]. Doppler can be used to analyse hypoechoic lesions which pose a "cystic or solid" problem. The presence of vascularisation in an echogenic lesion indicates that the lesion is tissue. However, the absence of vascularisation does not rule out the presence of a tissue portion [5] (fig. 6).

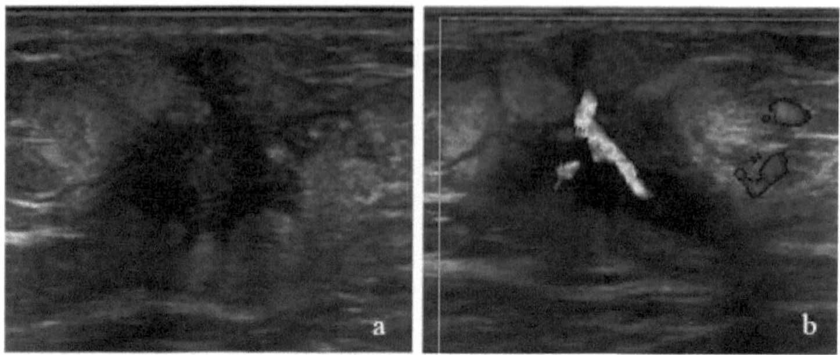

Fig. 6 Doppler mode (a) B-mode ultrasound. Hypoechoic mass with spiculated contours, (b) Doppler mode ultrasound. Intralesional vascularisation.

3.5. Elastography

Elastography is a non-invasive technique used in conjunction with ultrasound qualitatively, semi-quantitatively or quantitatively assess the deformability of lesions subjected to stress [16, 17]. The image obtained is then translated into an elastogram. This technique was developed to improve the specificity of B-mode breast ultrasound by adding compressibility and lesion "hardness" to the criteria of echostructure and lesion morphology (fig. 7). Breast elastography uses two distinct modes: free-hand elastography and shear-wave elastography.

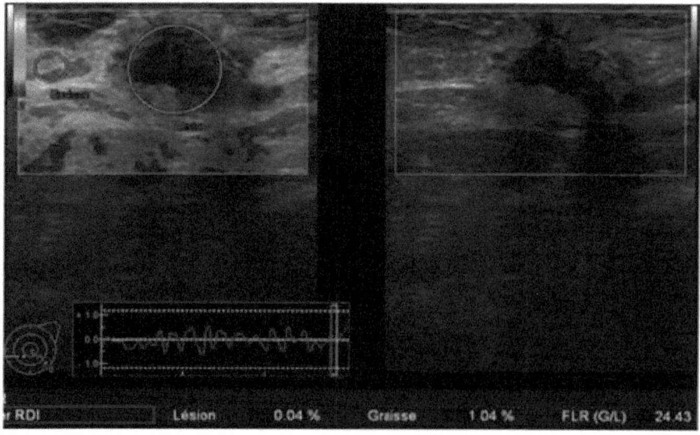

Fig. 7: Elastography. Elastography. Calculation of the elasticity ratio in standard deviation.

4. Ultrasound [18-24]

Several ultrasound aspects are encountered, depending on the proportion of adipose tissue, fibroglandular tissue and ductal elements. The appearance may also vary according to the glandular sector being analysed. In adult women, we find the following elements from surface to depth:

4.1. The skin covering

The thickness of the skin varies from 0.5 to 2 mm. It is visualised on ultrasound as a double echogenic line separated by a fine hypoechoic border (fig. 8). These lines merge at the nipple-areolar plate.

4.2. The nipple

The nipple is a hypoechoic structure which may be responsible for attenuation of ultrasound, in which case it is necessary to obliquely position the probe to explore the retroareolar region (fig. 8).

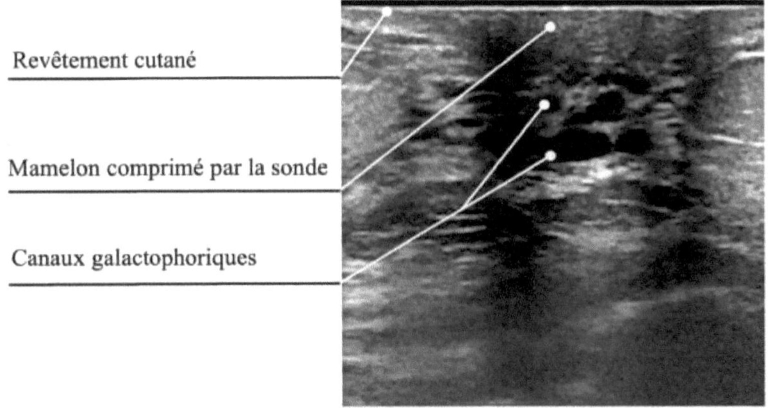

Fig. 8: Ultrasound section centred on the nipple.

4.3. Glandular tissue

The echogenicity of glandular parenchyma varies with age and individual composition. In young women and during pregnancy and lactation, the glandular tissue is often hypoechoic and homogeneous; during periods of genital activity, the glandular parenchyma is hyperechoic and homogeneous, of variable thickness (fig. 9). With age, the mammary parenchyma becomes heterogeneous due to fatty involution, the echostructure is hypoechoic interspersed with hyperechoic areas corresponding to connective fibres and residual parenchyma. When fibrous involution predominates, the echostructure is hyperechoic and heterogeneous.

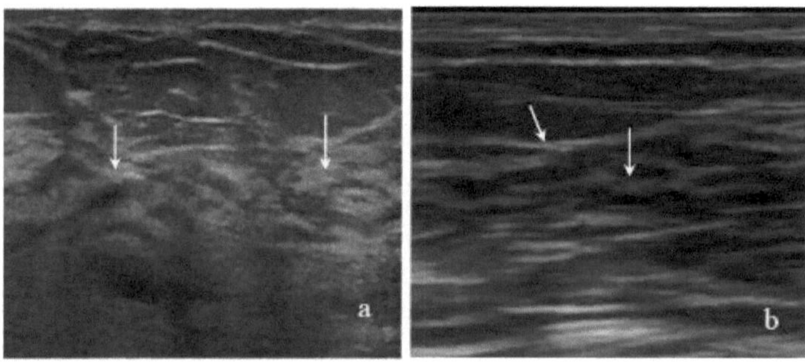

Fig. 9 Glandular parenchyma on ultrasound (a) Glandular tissue hyperechoic (arrows). (b) Glandular tissue in fat involution (arrows),

4.4. Connective tissue

The connective tissue is hyperechoic, often confused with glandular tissue. Cooper's ligaments are hyperechoic, passing through the layer of subcutaneous fatty tissue and appearing as thin, uniformly echogenic bands (fig. 10).

4.5. Adipose tissue

The subcutaneous fat appears as a hypoechoic line of variable thickness, divided by triangular hyperechoic structures representing Duret's ridges, the attachment zone of Cooper's ligaments. Intraglandular fatty tissue appears as well-limited oblong hypoechoic areas. In dorsal recumbency, the thickness of the retromammary fatty space is reduced in contrast to the mammographic appearance. This fatty space appears as a homogeneous hypoechoic band (fig. 10).

4.6. The muscles

The muscle planes appear as echogenic lamellar structures (fig. 10).

4.7. Ribs

The ribs are seen as hyperechoic, attenuating arciform structures (fig. 10).

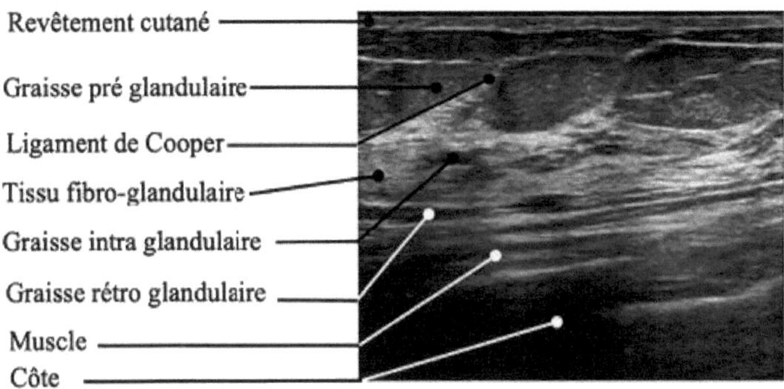

Fig. 10. Constitution of the breast. Ultrasound scan.

4.8. Vessels

Axillary vessels appear as hypoechoic tubular structures. They are best analysed in Doppler mode. Intra mammary vessels are sometimes visible in Doppler mode (fig. 11).

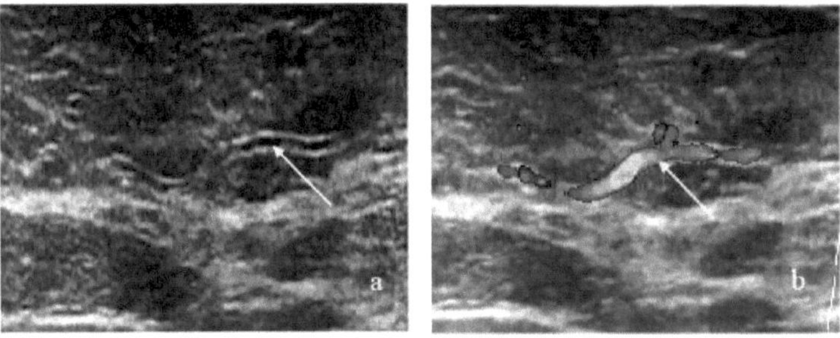

Fig. 11 Intramammary vessels. (a) Ultrasound. Tubular structure

4.9. Lymphatic vessels

Lymphatic vessels are absent in a normal breast. The lymph nodes appear as a kidney-shaped or coffee-bean-shaped structure with a hypoechoic cortex and a hyperechoic fatty hilum (fig. 12).

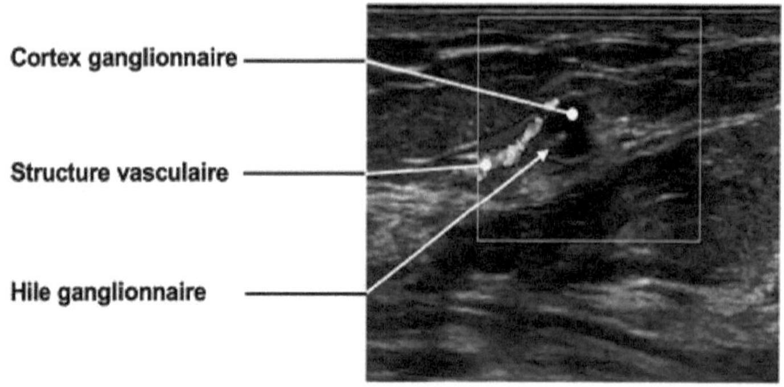

Fig. 12 Intramammary ganglion. Doppler ultrasound. Hypoechoic lymph node cortex and hyperechoic fatty lymph node hilum in a vascular pathway.

CHAPTER III

BI-RADS Glossary

1. Echo structure assessment

The ACR BI-RADS classification describes three basic types of echostructure (fig. 13):

- type a: homogeneous fatty echostructure with fat lobules and echogenic bands of Cooper's ligaments, with no echogenic zone in the area analysed ;
- type b: uniformly echogenic homogeneous fibroglandular ;
- type c: heterogeneous fibroglandular, the heterogeneity may be focal or diffuse.

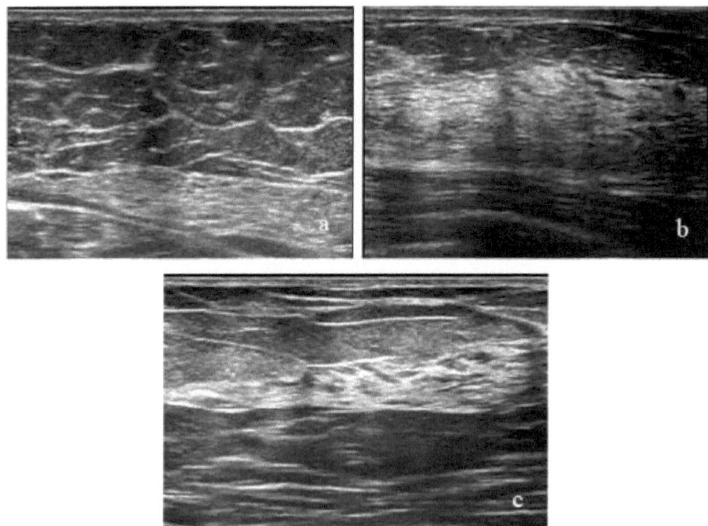

Fig. 13 Echostructure according to the ACR BI-RADS lexicon. Ultrasound.
(a) Homogeneous fat echostructure. (b) Homogeneous fibroglandular echostructure. (c) heterogeneous echostructure (focal or diffuse).

2. Description of lesions according to the BI-RADS lexicon

2.1. Weights

In ultrasound, a mass must be visible in two orthogonal views, in the form of a nodular lesion. The BI-RADS lexicon criteria for analysis a mass are: shape, orientation in relation to the skin, contours, interface, echostructures, posterior acoustic effects.

2.1.1. Shape

The shape can be :

- **Oval**: an ellipsoid or ovoid mass (fig. 14).
- **Round:** a spherical, ball-shaped, circular or globular mass (fig. 15).
- **Irregular:** a mass whose shape is neither round nor oval (fig. 16).

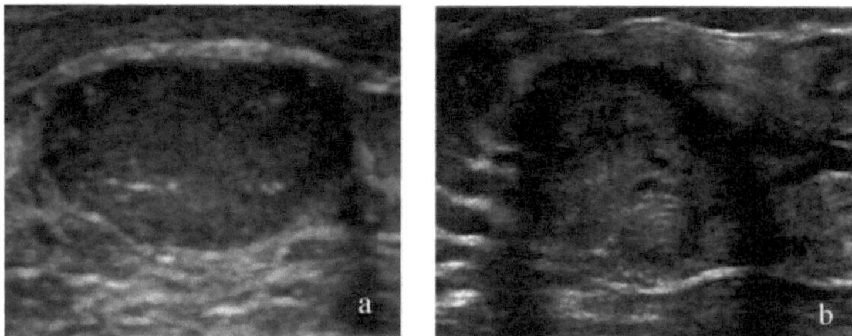

Fig. 14. Oval shape. (a) Fibroadenoma. (b) Mucinous carcinoma.

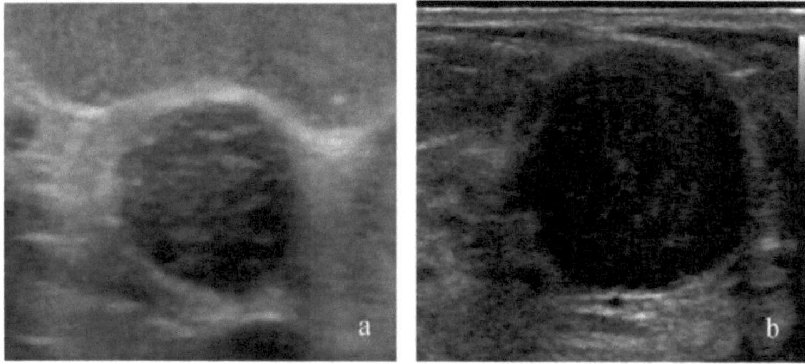

Fig. 15. Round shape. (a+b) Fibroadenoma.

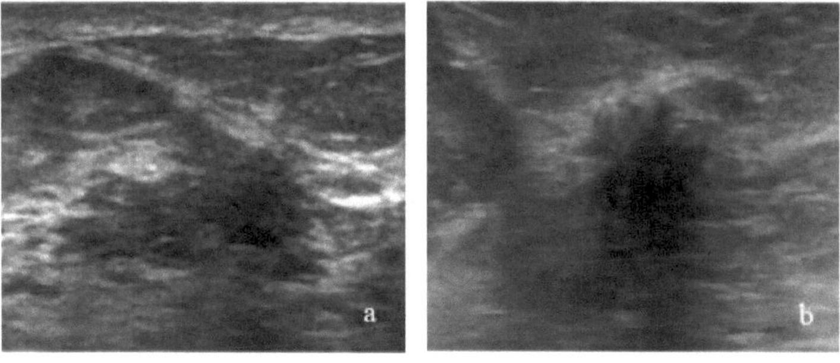

Fig. 16. Irregular shape. (a) Adenosis (b) Non-specific infiltrating carcinoma.

2.1.2. Orientation in relation to the skin

Some benign masses have a horizontal orientation, wider than high, although many cancers have this orientation. Conversely, benign masses almost never develop vertically (perpendicularly) (fig. 17,18).

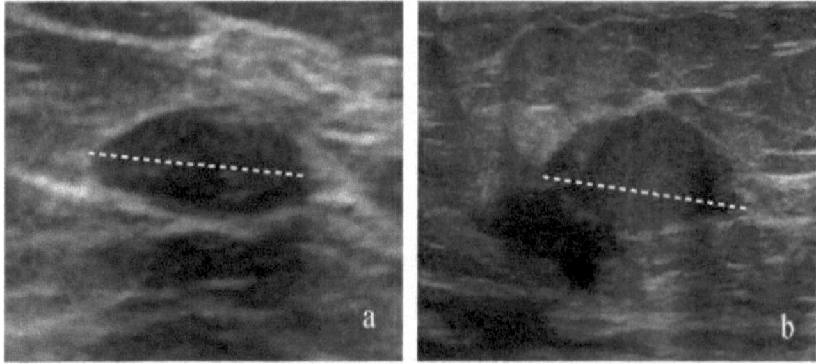

Fig. 17. Orientation of the mass. Parallel to the skin. (a) Fibroadenoma. (b) Micropapillary carcinoma.

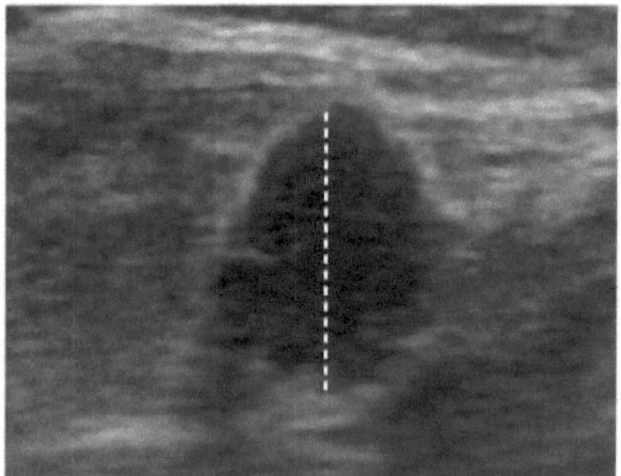

Fig. 18. Orientation of the mass. Not parallel to the skin. Vertical long axis. Papillary carcinoma.

2.1.3. Contours

- **Circumscribed:** sharp contours on at least 75% of the edges (fig. 19).
- **Non-circumscribed :**
- **Microlobulated** when the lobulations are very small, between 1 and 2 mm, and numerous, greater than 3 (fig. 20).

- **Indistinct** when the boundaries of the mass with adjacent tissue are not defined (fig. 21).
- **Angular** when the boundaries of the mass form angles that are usually acuteê (fig. 22).
- **Spiculated** when the mass has hypoechoic extensions (fig. 23).

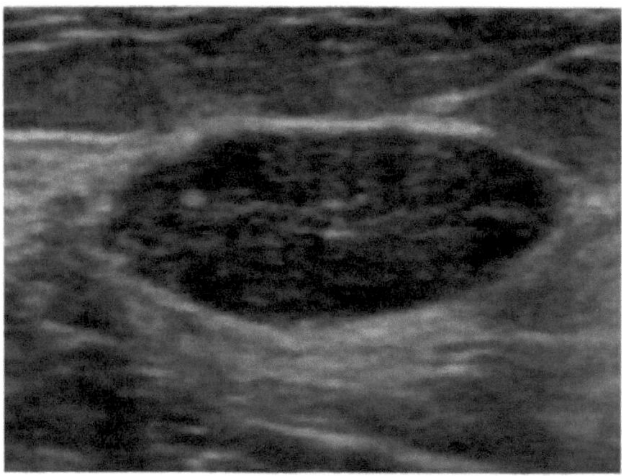

Fig. 19. Circumscribed contours. Clear contours visible around the entire circumference of the mass. Fibroadenoma.

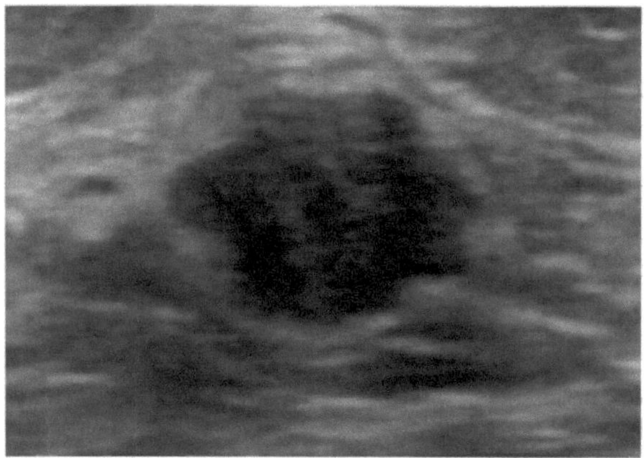

Fig. 20. Microlobulated outline. Small lobulations, more than 3. Phyllodes tumour.

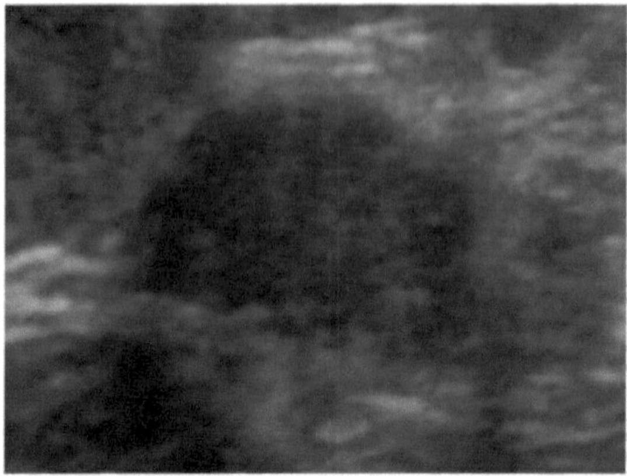

Fig. 21. indistinct contours. Boundaries with adjacent tissue are blurred. Cancer.

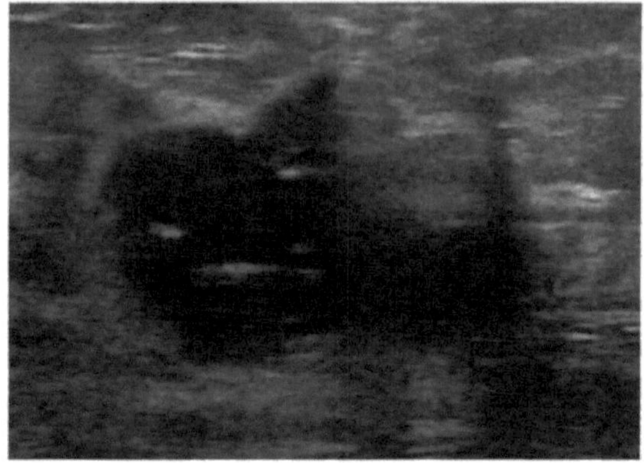

Fig. 22. Angular contours. The boundaries of the mass form acute angles. Cancer.

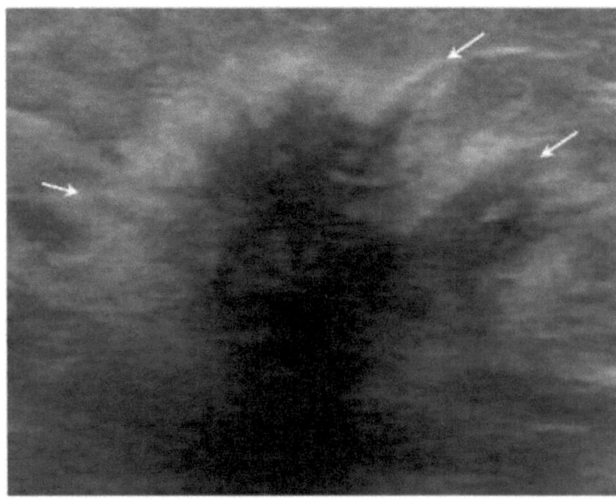

Fig. 23. Spiculated contours. The mass shows hypoechoic extensions (arrows). Cancer.

2.1.4. Interface or transition zone

Presence or absence of a thin echogenic line (capsule) (fig. 24) or a thick peripheral echogenic halo, generally found in certain cancers and abscesses (fig. 25).

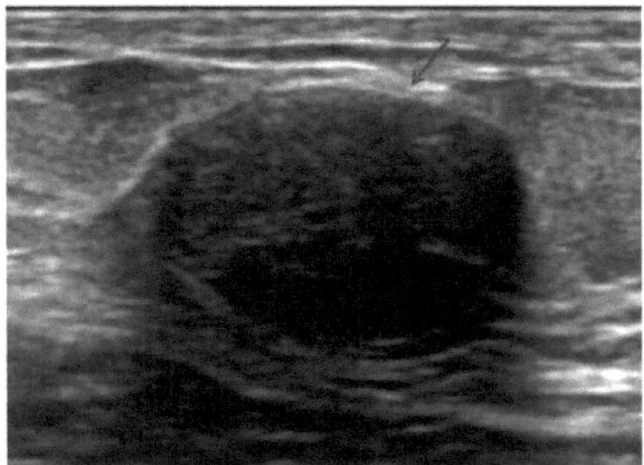

Fig. 24. Fine interface. Presence of an echogenic line around the mass (arrow). Fibroadenoma.

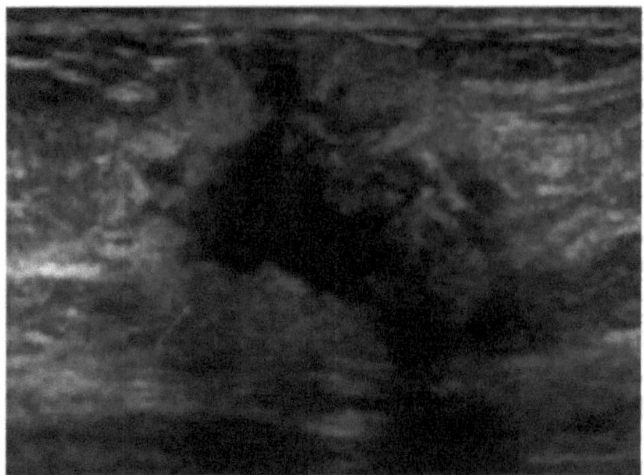

Fig. 25. Thick interface. Thick peripheral echogenic halo (arrow).

2.1.5. Echostructures

The echostructure must be assessed in comparison with that of the fat. It may be anechogenic, hypoechoic, isoechoic, hyperechoic (more echogenic than fat), complex (cystic and solid) or heterogeneous (figs. 26, 27, 28, 29, 30, 31).

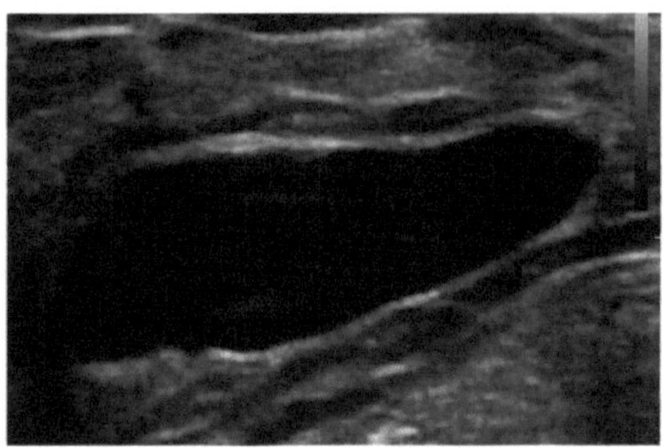

Fig. 26. Anechoic echostructure. Cyst.

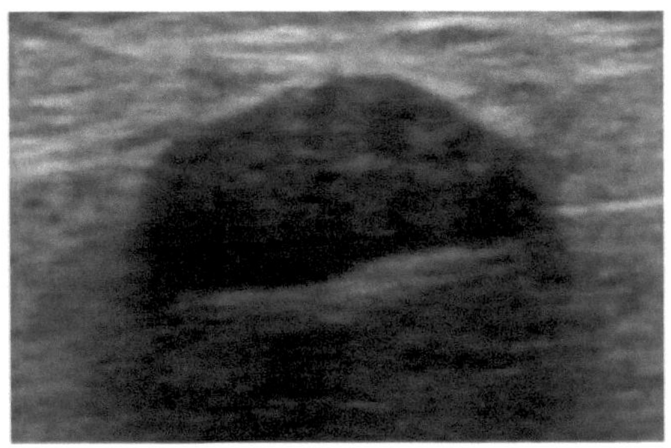

Fig. 27. Hypoechoic echostructure. Fibroadenoma.

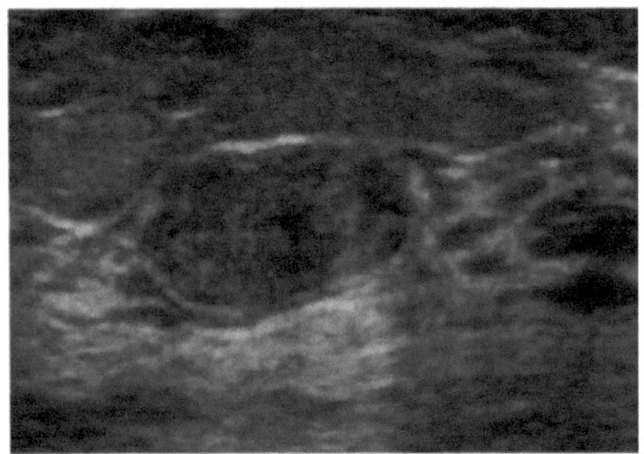

Fig. 28. Isoechogenic echostructure. Fibroadenoma.

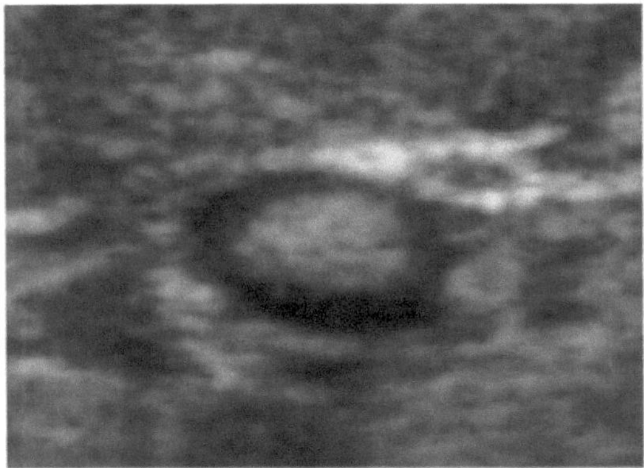

Fig. 29. Hyperechoic echostructure. Fibrocystic mastopathy.

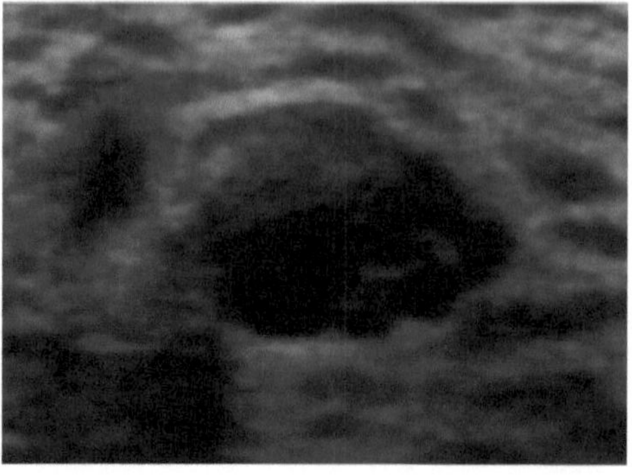

Fig. 30. Complex echostructure. Fibrocystic mastopathy.

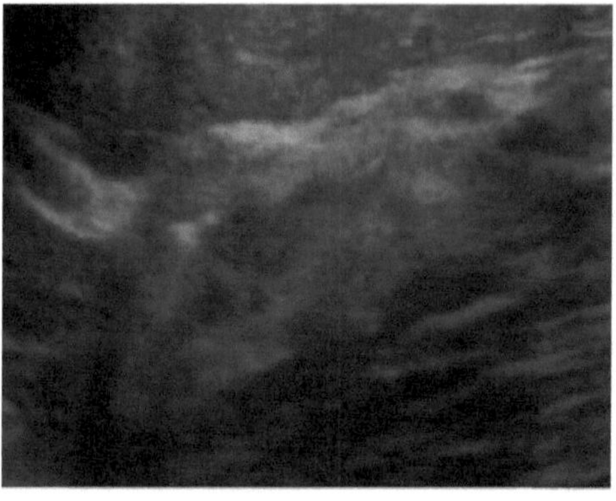

Fig. 31. Heterogeneous echostructure. Invasive lobar carcinoma.

2.1.6. Acoustic after-effects

The posterior acoustic bundle can be :

- unmodified (no subsequent acoustic effect) (fig. 32) ;
- reinforced (posterior reinforcement) (fig. 33) ;
- totally or partially attenuated (posterior attenuation) (fig. 34) ;
- mixed, combining a strengthening of the ultrasound beam and posterior attenuation (mixed effects) (fig. 35).

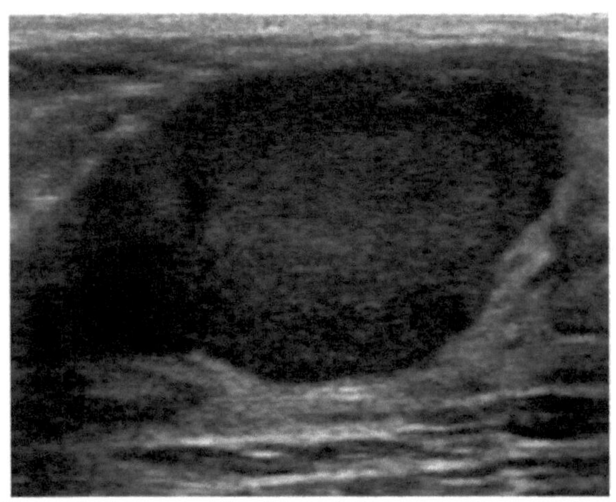

Fig. 32. Posterior acoustic signs of the mass. No posterior effect. Fibroadenoma.

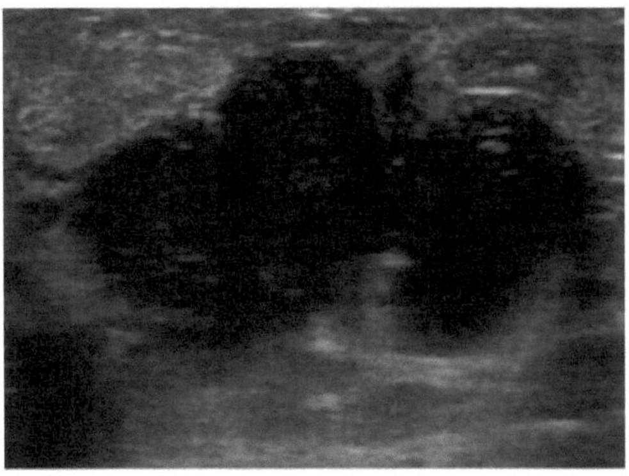

Fig. 33. Posterior acoustic signs of the mass. Reinforcement posterior acoustic (asterisk). Cancer.

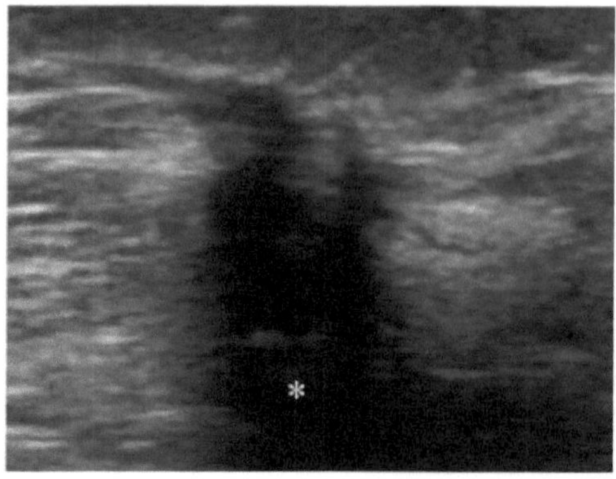

Fig. 34. Posterior acoustic signs of the mass. Attenuation posterior (asterisk). Cancer.

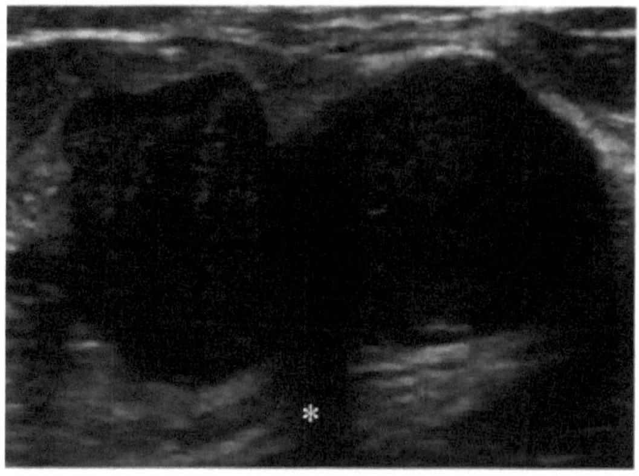

Fig. 35. Posterior acoustic signs of the mass. Combined effects, posterior attenuation (white asterisk) and enhancement (red asterisk). Fibroadenoma.

2.2. Calcifications

Calcifications are easily visible on ultrasound with a high-frequency linear probe, especially if they are located in a hypoechoic mass (fig. 36, 37). Calcifications outside a mass are usually less suspicious.

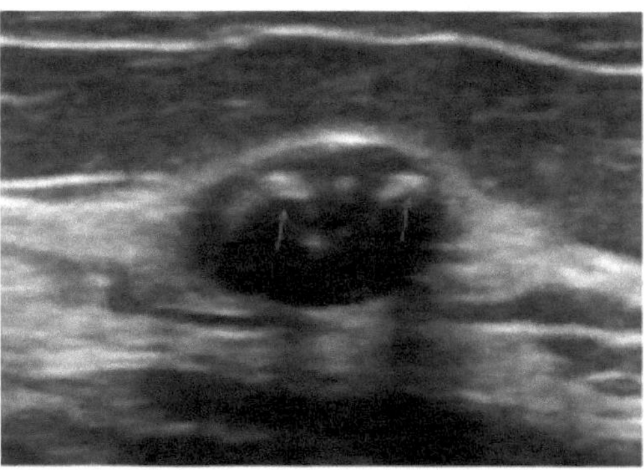

Fig. 36. Calcifications in the mass (arrows). Fibroadenoma

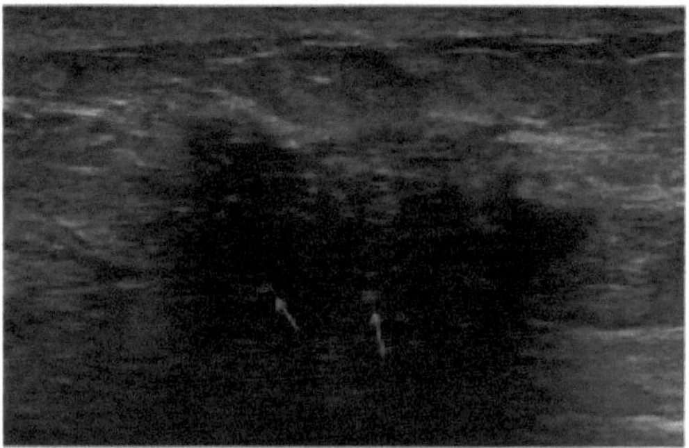

Fig. 37. Calcifications in the mass (arrows). Carcinoma infiltrating root canal.

2.3. Associated signs

Associated signs may be related to the effect a mass on the tissues, such as architectural disorganisation, ectasia or ductal deformities, skin changes (thickening, retraction) or redema (fig. 38, 39).

The vascularisation of a mass using colour or energy Doppler should also be analysed, and may be absent, increased, peripheral, central or irregular in a malignant lesion (fig. 41).

Elastography is used to assess the hardness of lesions. The mass may be soft or deformable, of intermediate hardness, rigid or only slightly deformable (fig. 41).

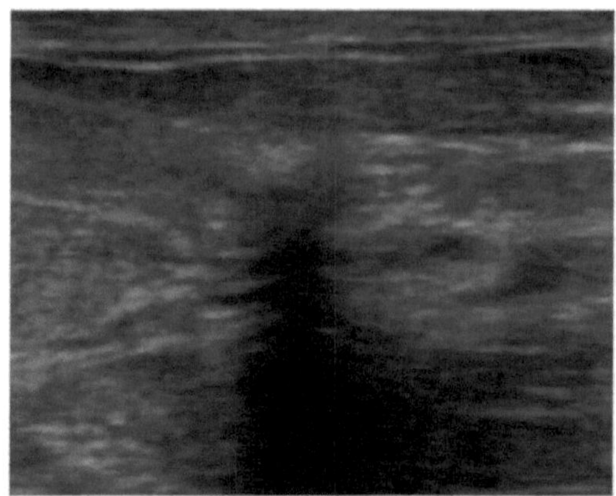
Fig. 38. Architectural disorganisation.

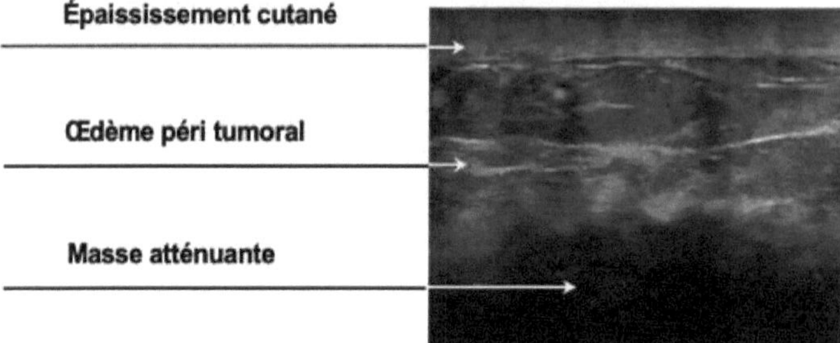

Fig. 39. Associated signs of a malignant mass.

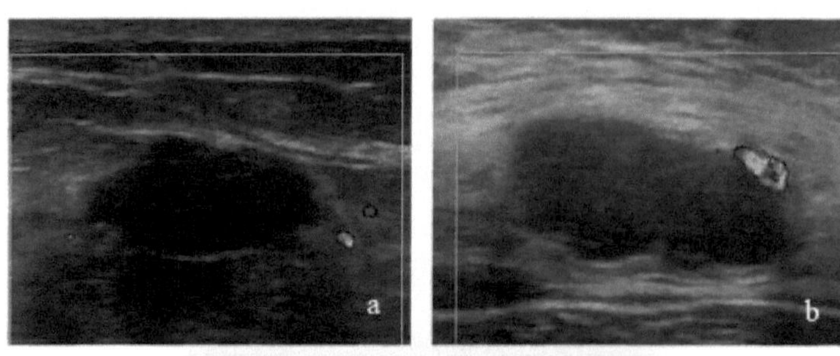

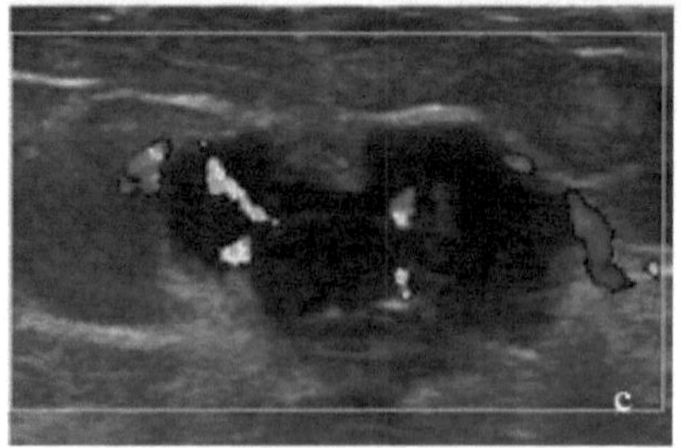

Fig. 40. Vascularisation of the mass (a) No vascularisation. Fibroadenoma. (b) Peripheral vascularisation. Fibroadenoma. (c) Irregular central and peripheral vascularisation. Non-specific infiltrating carcinoma.

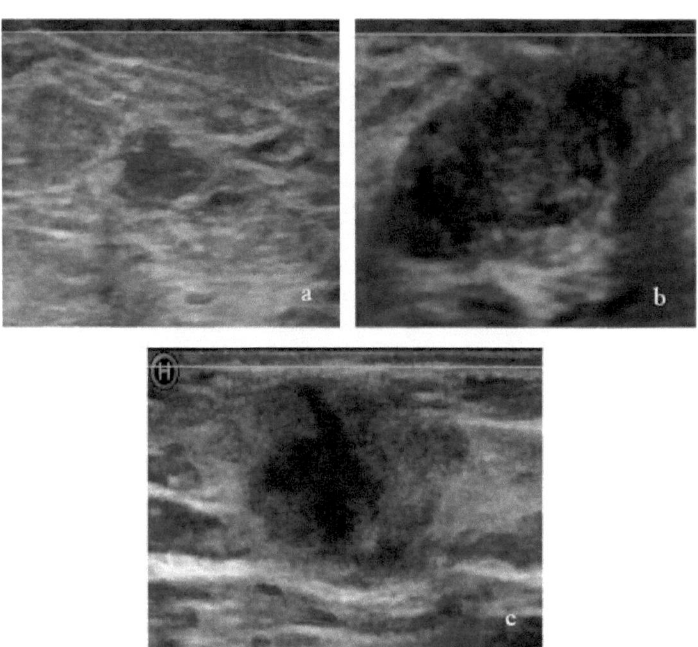

Fig. 41. Elastography. Mass (a) Soft. Fibroadenoma. (b) Intermediate hardness. Fibroadenoma. (c) Rigid. Non-specific infiltrating carcinoma.

2.4. Special cases according to BI-RADS

Some cases are fairly typical in ultrasound. These are simple cysts, contiguous microcysts, complicated cysts (echogenic), skin masses, foreign bodies and implants, intra-mammary and axillary lymph nodes, vascular anomalies (venous thrombosis), postoperative collections and scars, cytosteatonecrosis (figs. 42, 43, 44, 45, 46 and 47).

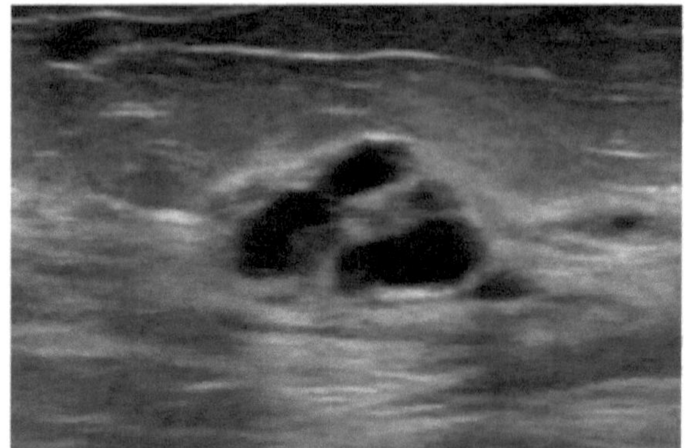

Fig. 42. Special cases. Clusters of microcysts.

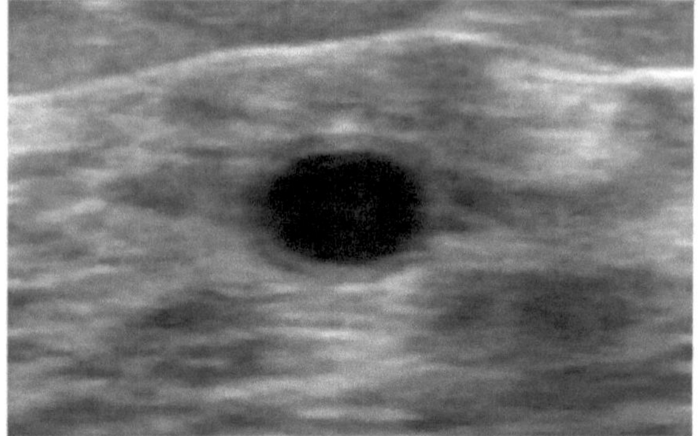

Fig. 43. Special cases. Complicated cyst.

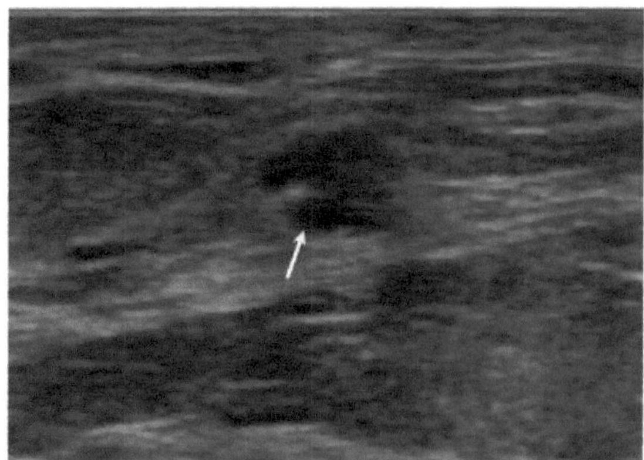

Fig. 44. Special cases. Intramammary ganglion (arrow).

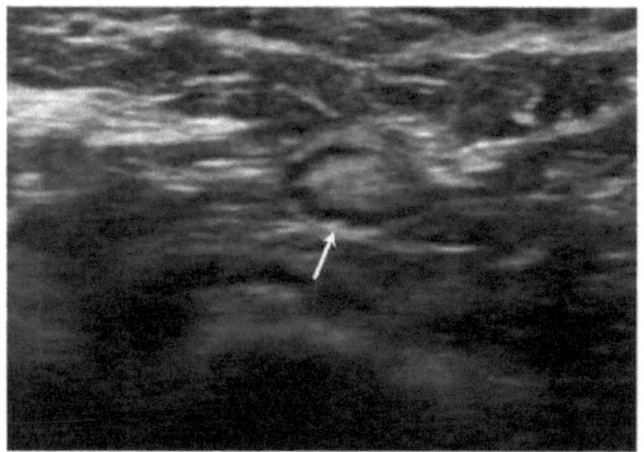

Fig. 45. Special cases. Axillary ganglion (arrow).

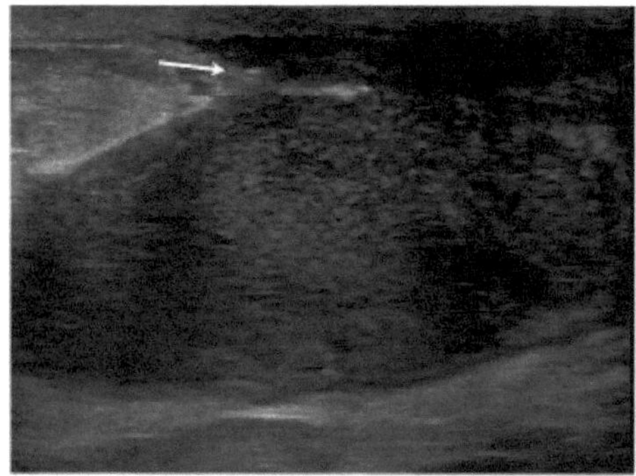

Fig. 46. Special cases. Abscessed collection, showing a cutaneous disruption (arrow).

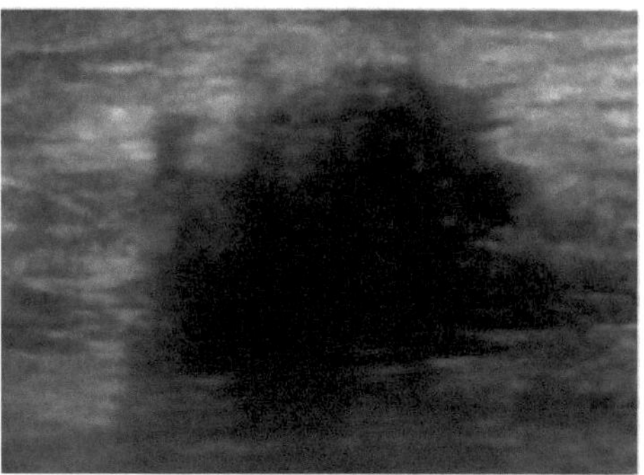

Fig. 47. Special cases. Cytosteatonecrosis.

3. Locating a lesion

Lesions should be located according to side, quadrant, hourly radius and distance from the nipple in cm. The use of the hourly radius helps to avoid errors regarding the side of the breast, given that the radii are different on the two breasts, for example a lesion on the right QSE is located at 10H on the right and 2H on the left. As on mammography, a central lesion is located behind the nipple, a retro-areolar lesion is located in the central part of the anterior third of the breast and a lesion of the axillary extension in the upper part of the QSE. For these three particular areas, it is not necessary to use the hourly radius or the quadrant (fig. 48).

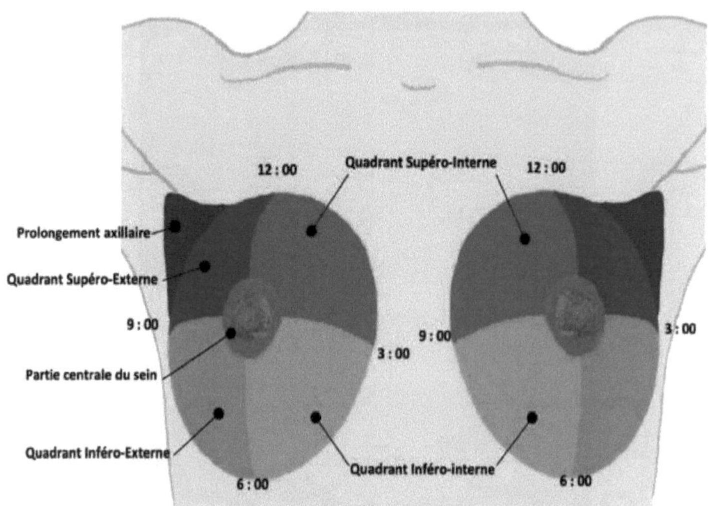

Fig. 48. Hourly quadrants of the breast.

4. Probability of malignancy score

The BI-RADS 0 category is reserved only for incomplete examinations, and additional mammography is requested after the ultrasound or previous images not available on the day of the ultrasound examination for comparison.

BI-RADS 1 or 2 categories, benign anomalies.

The BI-RADS 3 category always reflects an anomaly that is probably benign requiring short-term monitoring, with a probability of malignancy of between 0 and 2%. Three types of ultrasound anomaly can be found in the BI-RADS 3 category:

- benign solid mass (oval shape, regular contours, homogeneous echostructure, parallel orientation, posterior enhancement) (fig. 49) ;
- complicated, homogeneous echogenic cysts (0.3% risk of malignancy) (fig. 50) ;
- clusters of microcysts (fig. 42).

Three other entities can be classified as BI-RADS 3 :

- post-surgical distortion;
- doubt about a true or pseudo nodule in the case of a fatty lobule;
- a hyperechoic mass with a hypoechoic or anechoic centre associated with cytosteatonecrosis (fig. 51).

Monitoring of an anomaly classified as BI-RADS 3 on ultrasound is as follows: check-up at 4 months of the breast carrying the anomaly, check-up at 1 year, then check-up at 2 or even 3 years. If the anomaly is stable at 2 or 3 years, it is reclassified as BI-RADS 2.

The BI-RADS 4 classification means the existence of an undetermined abnormality requiring biopsy. The PPV of BI-RADS 4 cancer is broad, between 2% and 95%, and it is recommended that the sub-categories BI-RADS 4a, BI-RADS 4b and BI-RADS 4c be used (figs. 52, 53, 54, 55, 56, 57, 58).

A BI-RADS 4a lesion has a positive predictive value for cancer of between 2 and 10%. A lesion classified as BI-RADS 4b has a positive predictive value of 10 to 50% for cancer. A BI-RADS 4c lesion has a positive predictive value for cancer of 50 to 95%.

A BI-RADS 5 lesion is suggestive of cancer with a PPV greater than 95% (figs. 59, 60, 61, 62); a biopsy must be taken obtain a histological diagnosis.

BI-RADS 6 means proven cancer.

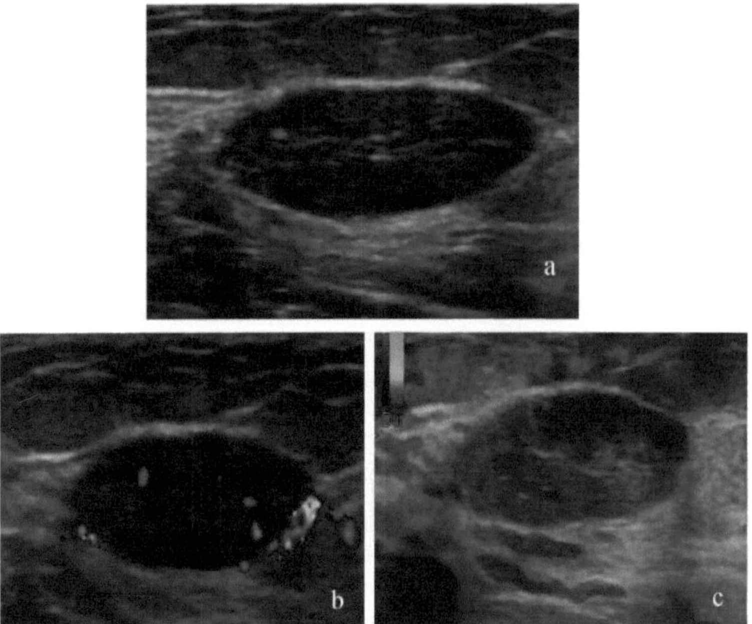

Fig. 49. Masses classified as BI-RADS 3. (a) B-mode ultrasound. Oval mass, oriented parallel to the skin, circumscribed contours, fine interface, hypoechoic, homogeneous and without posterior acoustic effect. (b) Colour Doppler. Poorly vascularised mass. (c) Elastography. Soft lesion. Fibroadenoma.

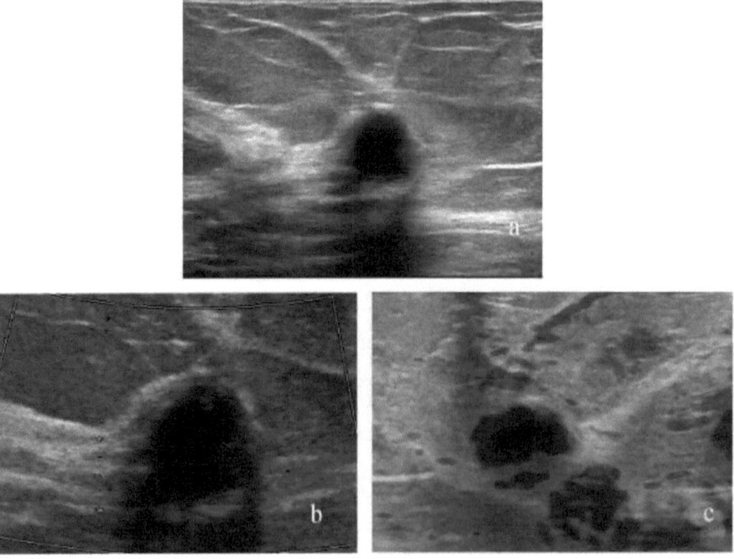

Fig. 50. Masses classified as BI-RADS 3. (a) B-mode ultrasound. Round mass, oriented parallel to the skin, circumscribed contours, fine interface, hypoechoic, homogeneous and without posterior acoustic effect. (b) Colour Doppler. Non-vascularised. (c) Elastography. Blue-green-red artefact at the level of the lesion testifies to its cystic nature. Inflammatory cyst.

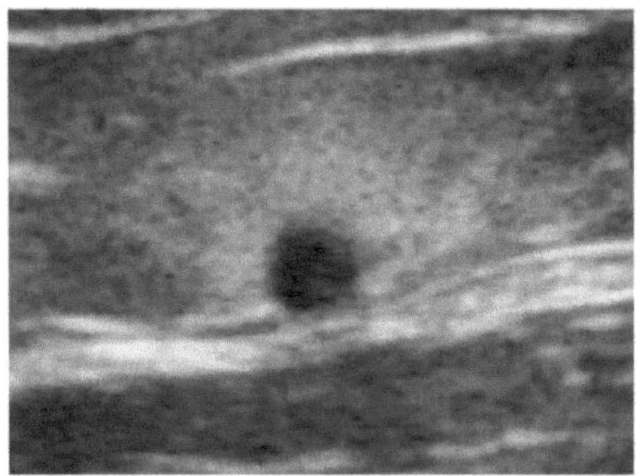

Fig. 51. Masses classified as BI-RADS 3. B-mode ultrasound. Hyperechoic mass with hypoechoic centre. Cytosteatonecrosis.

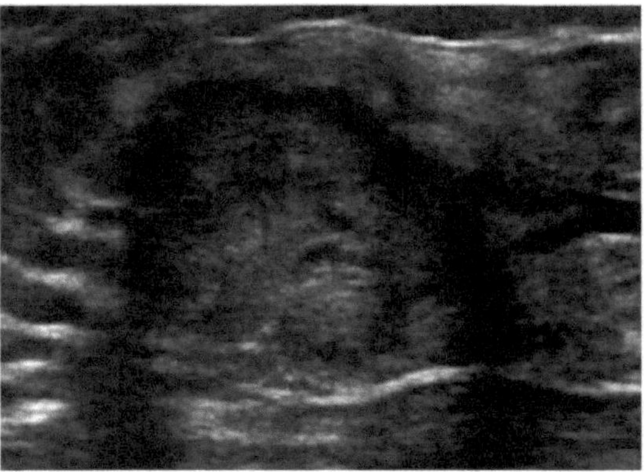

Fig. 52. Masses classified as BI-RADS 4a. Oval mass, parallel to the skin, microlobulated contours, thin interface, hypoechoic, discreetly heterogeneous and without posterior acoustic effect. Mucinous carcinoma.

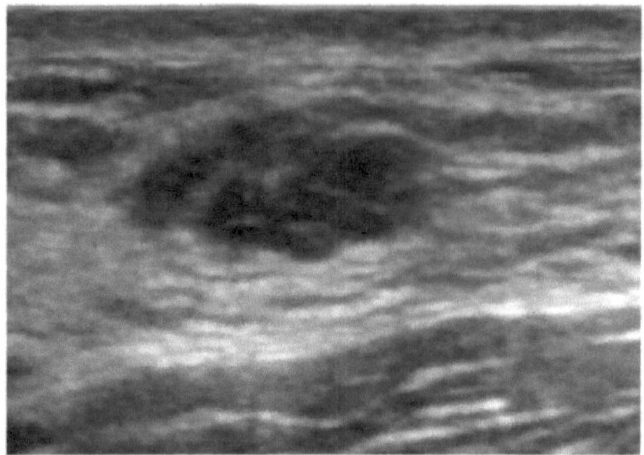

Fig. 53. Masses classified as BI-RADS 4a. Oval mass, parallel to the skin, microlobulated contours, thin interface, hypoechoic, discreetly heterogeneous and without posterior acoustic effect. Fibroadenoma.

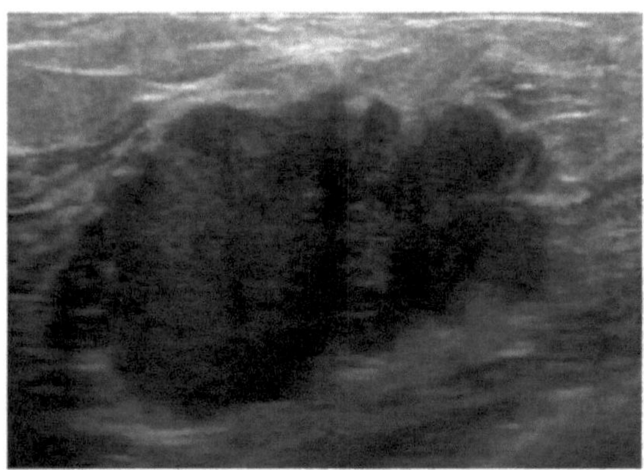

Fig. 54. Masses classified as BI-RADS 4b. Oval mass, parallel to the skin, microlobulated contours, thin interface, strongly hypoechoic, heterogeneous and without posterior acoustic effect. Non-specific infiltrating carcinoma.

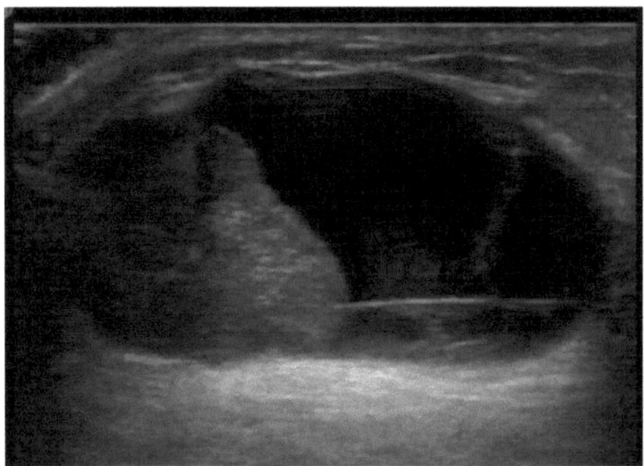

Fig. 55. Masses classified as BI-RADS 4b. Complex solid-cystic mass, the solid portion of which presents with a mural nodule (asterisk), hypoechoic, with microlobulated contours and the thick-walled cystic portion containing echoes and declining debris within it. Intracystic papillary carcinoma.

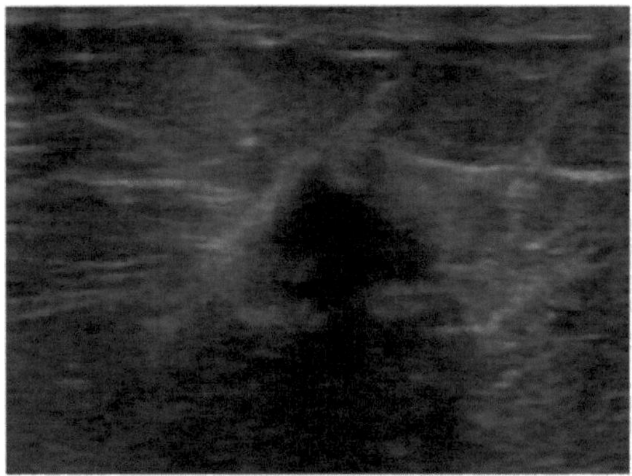

Fig. 56. Masses classified as BI-RADS 4c. Irregularly shaped mass, parallel to the skin, with indistinct contours and a thin interface with posterior attenuation. Invasive lobular carcinoma.

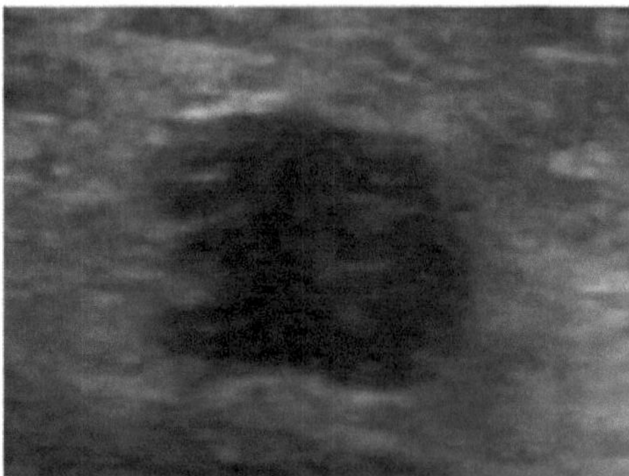

Fig. 57. Masses classified as BI-RADS 4c. Oval mass, not parallel to the skin, indistinct contours, thin interface, strongly hypoechoic and without posterior acoustic effect. Non-specific infiltrating carcinoma.

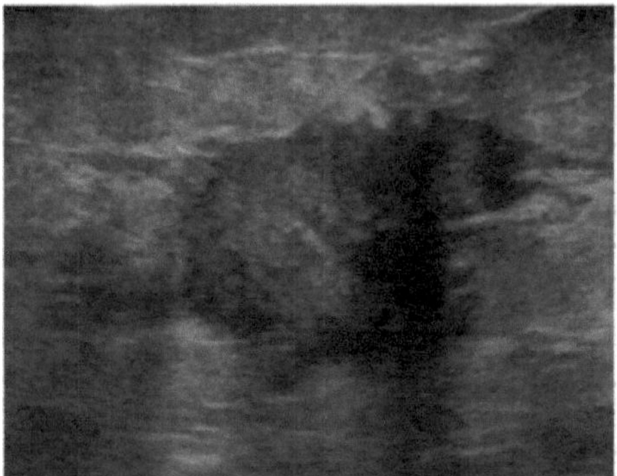

Fig. 58. Masses classified as BI-RADS 4c. Irregular mass, parallel to the skin, indistinct contours, thin interface, strongly hypoechoic and without posterior acoustic effect. Invasive apocrine carcinoma.

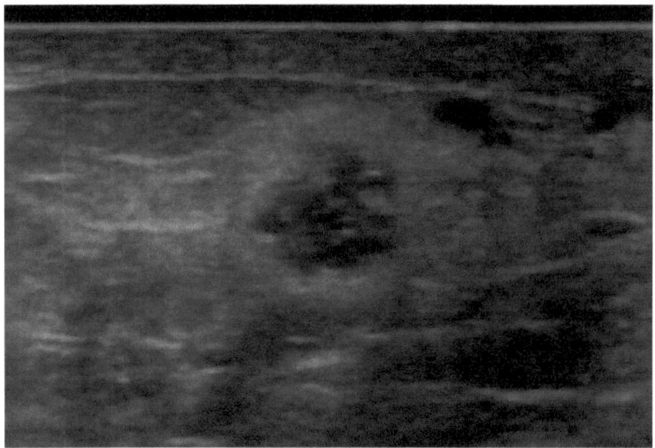

Fig. 59. Masses classified as BI-RADS 5. Irregular mass, not parallel to the skin, with angular contours, surrounded by a peripheral echogenic halo, hypoechoic and without posterior acoustic effect. Idiopatic granular mastitis.

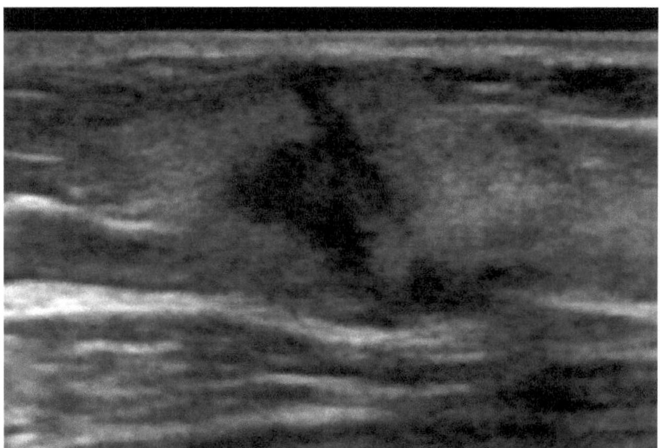

Fig. 60. Masses classified as BI-RADS 5. Irregular mass, not parallel to the skin, with angular contours, surrounded by a peripheral echogenic halo, hypoechoic and without posterior acoustic effect. Non-specific infiltrating carcinoma.

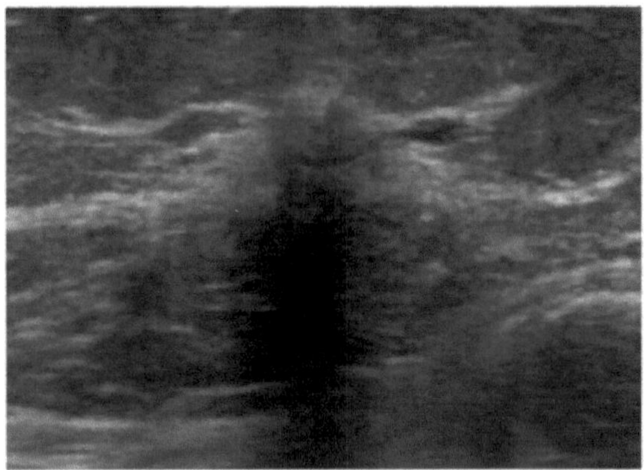

Fig. 61. Masses classified as BI-RADS 5. Irregular mass, orientation not parallel to the skin, spiculated contours, surrounded by a peripheral echogenic halo, hypoechoic and posterior acoustic attenuation. Non-specific infiltrating carcinoma.

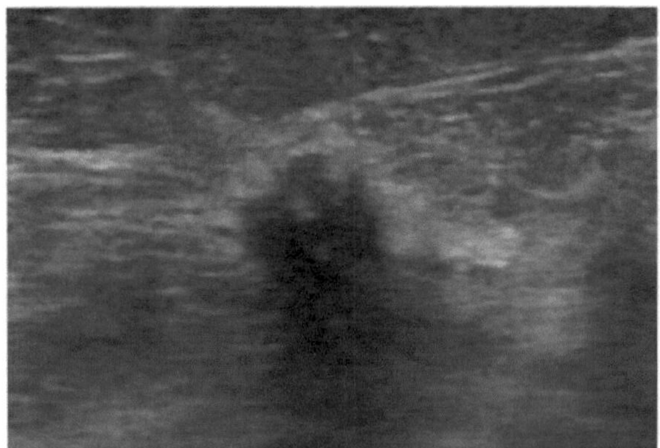

Fig. 62. Masses classified as BI-RADS 5. Irregular mass, orientation not parallel to the skin, spiculated contours, surrounded by a peripheral echogenic halo, hypoechoic, shows calcifications within it posterior acoustic attenuation. Non-specific infiltrating carcinoma.

References

1. D'Orsi CJ et al. ACR BI-RADS Atlas, Breast Imaging Reporting and Data System. Reston, VA, American College of Radiology; 2013.
2. Couturaud B, Fitoussi A. Anatomy / surgery of breast cancer. Conservative treatment, oncoplasty. Techniques chirurgicales gynécologie. Elsevier Masson; 2011; 4-7.
3. Corsetti V, Houssami N, Ferrari A, Ghirardi M, Bellarosa S, Angelini O, et al. Breast screening with ultrasound in women with mammography-negative dense breasts: evidence on incremental cancer detection and false positives, and associated cost. Eur J Cancer. 2008 Mar;44(4):539-44.
4. Athanasiou A, Tardivon A, Ollivier L, Thibault F, El Khoury C, Neuenschwander S. How to optimize breast ultrasound. Eur J Radiol. 2009 Jan;69(1):6-13.
5. Weinstein SP, Conant EF, Sehgal C. Technical advances in breast ultrasound imaging. Semin Ultrasound CT MR. 2006 Aug;27(4):273-83.
6. Sehgal CM, Weinstein SP, Arger PH, Conant EF. A review of breast ultrasound. J Mammary Gland Biol Neoplasia. 2006 Apr;11(2):113-23.
7. Amersham Health. Encyclopaedia of Medical Imaging. http://eu.aershamhealth/com/medcyclopaedia/
8. Clevert DA, Jung EM, Jungius KP, Ertan K, Kubale R. Value of tissue harmonic imaging (THI) and contrast harmonic imaging (CHI) in detection and characterisation of breast tumours. Eur Radiol 2007 ; 17 : 1-10.
9. Rosen EL, Soo MS. Tissue harmonic imaging sonography of breast lesions: improved margin analysis, conspicuity, and image quality compared to conventional ultrasound. Clin Imaging. 2001 Nov-Dec;25(6):379-84.
10. Athanasiou A, Balleyguier C. New techniques in breast ultrasound. Imagerie de la Femme. 2007;17(4):247-54.
11. Huber S, Wagner M, Medl M, Czembirek H. Real-time spatial compound imaging in breast ultrasound. Ultrasound Med Biol 2002; 28: 155-63.
12. Cha JH, Moon WK, Cho N, Chung SY, Park SH, Park JM, et al.

differentiation of benign from malignant solid breast masses: conventional US versus compound imaging. Radiology 2005;237:841-6.

13. Balu-Maestro C. Basics of breast ultrasound. Imager ie du sein. Paris : Elsevier-Masson ; 2012. p. 101-17.

14. Dickinson RJ, Hill CR. Measurement of soft tissue motion using correlation between A-scans.Ultrasound Med Biol 1982;8(3):263-71.

15. Krouskop TA, Dougherty DR, Vinson FS. A pulsed Doppler ultrasonic system for making noninvasive measurements of the mechanical properties of soft tissue. J Rehabil Res Dev 1987;24(2):1-8.

16. Youk JH, Gweon HM, Son EJ. Shear-wave elastography in breast ultrasonography: the state of the art. Ultrasonography. 2017 Oct;36(4):300-309. doi: 10.14366/usg.17024.

17. Tristant H, Benmussa M, Bokobsa J, Elbaz P. Variation of the normal breast: mammographic and ultrasonographic aspects. Encycl Méd Chir 1994; 810-G-15.

18. Levy L. The normal breast and its variants: breast cancers. Mammography and Mammary Ultrasound 2006.

19. Cartier JM, Bourjat P. The normal breast. Imagerie du sein : La pratique sénologique quotidienne 1998 ; 33-35.

20. Heywang-Kobrunner S H, Schreer I, Bassler R, Perlet C, Viehweg P. Normal breast. Imagerie diagnostique du sein : Mammographie, échographie, IRM, techniques interventionnelles 2007 ; 183-202.

21. Goumot PA, Bremond A, Dilhuydy MH, et al. La lecture mammographique : Sémiologie le sein normal. Le Sein : Son Image 1993.

22. Jokich PM, Monticciolo DL, Adler YT. Breast ultrasonography. Radiol Clin North Am 1992; 30: 993-1009.

23. Michelin J, Levy L. Normal breast and its variants: Diagnostic and interventional breast ultrasound. Collection d'imagerie radiologique. Masson, 1999; 9-13.

24. Neel-Paprocki V. Echo-anatomical reminders. Le Sein, 1994; 4: 73-77.

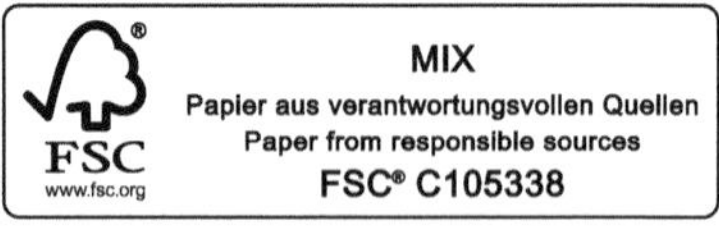

Printed by Books on Demand GmbH, Norderstedt / Germany